Kama Sutra

Step by step guided potions to connect deeply with your lover

By: Jessica Anderson.

© Copyright 2019 - All rights reserved

No part of this book may be reproduced in any form without permission in writing from the author. Reviewers may quote brief passages in reviews.

Table of Contents

Introduction 1
Chapter 1: What Is Kama Sutra? 4
   Background of Kama Sutra 5
   What does Kama Sutra talk about? 6
      Flirting and Courtship 6
      Intimacy and Foreplay 7
      Adultery 8
      Caste, Class 8
      Same-sex, Group-sex Relationships 9
Chapter 2: How can I Apply this to my Life in the Modern Day 10
   Preparing the Body 11
      Perfuming the Breath 12
      Bathing Together 12
      The Erogenous Zones 13
      Lips and Throats 13
      Best Foot Forward 14
   Sensual Skin 14
   Creating the Mood 15
      Flowers 16
      Soft Light 16
      Scenting the Room 16
      Champagne and Silk 16
      Perfuming the Skin 16
      Oil and Lotions 17
Chapter 3: How to Introduce Kama Sutra to the Bedroom in Today's World 18
   What is touching and caressing? 18

Embracing 19
    1. The First Group of Embrace 20
    2.   The Second Group of Embrace 22
    3.   Embracing Simple Members of the Body 24
Mutual Grooming 25

Chapter 4: How to use this to Deeply Connect with my Partner 27

Sensual Massage 27
The Basic Massaging Strokes 28
Using Massaging oil 30
Different Areas on the Body to Massage 31
Scratching 33
Hair Play 34

Chapter 5: Kissing and Mouthplay in the Bedroom in Today's World 36

Types of kissing 36
    The Bent Kiss 36
    The Turned Kiss 37
    The Straight Kiss 37
    Pressed Kiss 37
    Kissing the Upper Lips 38
    The Clasping Kiss 38
    A Young Girl's Kiss 38
Other ways to use kissing 39
    Kissing that kindles love 39
    Kissing that awakens 39
    Kissing that turns away 39
    Kissing the body 40
Biting 40
    The biting of a boar 40

The broken cloud 41
Cunnilingus 41
  Clitoral stimulation 41
  Stimulating the perineum 41
Fellatio 42
  Licking the Penis 42
  Butterfly flick 42

Chapter 6: Kama Sutra Sex Positions Explained **43**
  1. The Pressing Position 43
  2. The Mare's Position 44
  3. The Turning Position 45
  4. The Woman on Top Position 46
  5. The Yawning Position 46
  6. The Elephant Posture 47
  7. Level Feet Posture 48
  8. The Crab Embrace Position 48
  9. The Rainbow Arch Position 49
  10. Driving the Peg Home 50

Chapter 7: Before and After Sex **51**
What to do before sex by having a safer sex 51
  Non-Penetrative Sex 51
  Using Condoms 52
What to do after sex by prolonging the mood 52
  Rekindle the excitement 52
  Sustaining the harmony 53

Chapter 8: The Benefits of Kama Sutra **54**
  1. Kama Sutra values empowering women 54
  2. Kama Sutra makes a clear classification of a man's penis 54

3. Kama Sutra also emphasizes on living a healthy life and well-balanced one 55

4. Kama Sutra talks about enticing and approaching women . 55

5. Kama Sutra talks about eight different types of embrace ... 55

6. Kama Sutra teaches about kissing 55

7. Kama Sutra is divided into a set of 64 acts 56

8. Kama Sutra recommends that your scratch your partner 56

9. Kama Sutra recommends that your woman lover should reach orgasm first 56

10. Kama Sutra also talks about a woman's sex as being more than just sex penetrations 56

Chapter 9: How to Apply Everything you've Learnt about Kama Sutra 57

1. Approach your lover 57

2. Make an Attempt 57

3. Seduce 58

4. Go for any of the sex positions you've learned 58

5. Try an after sex fun 59

Conclusion 60

Introduction

Romance! Making love!! Sex!!! Call it what you want, but if you're no longer feeling that urge or satisfaction as much as you'd like, then there's going to be a problem. Believe it or not, most marriages that crashed, crashed because they are no longer getting the right satisfaction they want from the relationship. Men cheat on their wives because she doesn't please him anymore. Even women go out of their way to have a sexual partner that will make her feel that spark of romance.

Whatever the case may be, it wouldn't be fair to blame anybody. After all the people that cheat in their marriages or relationships do it with someone else. So, the big question is, what do they have that you don't?

Money? Beauty?

Yes, that counts at times. But the hidden truth is that the surest deal you can seal to keep your man or woman is in the bedroom. I'm not talking about just having a conversation. I'm talking about real hot, hardcore sex that would pop their brains out during orgasm. I bet you'd like to know-how. Well, keep reading!

Have you heard about Kama Sutra? If you have, then things just got a lot easier. If you haven't don't worry, you will get to catch the whole idea as we proceed. You see, a lot of people often don't get the entire concept of Kama Sutra. People think Kama Sutra is all about different sex position and that's all. You wouldn't be entirely wrong if you believe Kama Sutra is about sex positions. However, there's more to it than different sex positions.

Understanding the full benefits of Kama Sutra is one of the major things we'd be looking at in this book. Kama Sutra can help you in your relationship in ways you never thought possible. At times all that your partner needs is someone a little bit more emotional. You shouldn't have sex, like robots!

There was this scenario about a woman who no longer feels like having sex with her husband anymore. She claimed she no longer feels turned on by her husband. She further said all her husband does is to do a little talking, a little kissing and then he's in her, and under 5 minutes he's done and out leaving her completely unfulfilled. To the man, he believes they are having sex, but would you blame her if she cheats.

What about a scenario where a man finds it so difficult to make his woman have an orgasm. Smiles! Don't feel battered if you fall under this category it's one of those midlife crises common among men. Commonly, women don't have an orgasm as fast as men do. Is this true? Well, allow me to let you in on a little secret. Did you know that with the right foreplay and sex position you can make you woman have an orgasm in around 5-10 minutes?

It would interest you to know that Kama Sutra embraces a man approaching and enticing a woman. So, when you want to create that spark of emotion in your woman, there are specific steps you are supposed to take. I'd show you that as we proceed in the book. There are ways a man is supposed to touch a woman to express his desire to have sex with her. There are also ways a woman would react to the approach that would lead the man on further.

Kama Sutra talks about the different types of embrace which we'd be looking at in the book. Then there's also the vital kissing part, which you should do correctly. And of course the sexual-arts, which is an essential part. In all, Kama Sutra talks about sexuality at large.

Did you know that Kama Sutra values women with knowledge? I bet you didn't know that. Our society often ignores the fact that a woman needs to learn how to please her man before getting married. If a woman can learn the different forms of arts, including learning an instrument, solving a puzzle, laying a bed or even playing a word game, it would help her manage her husband and home properly. So, Kama Sutra encourages a woman to be knowledgeable.

Under no circumstance should you have a boring sexual life? Enhance your pleasure nerve and get that ultimate climax you've been craving with Kama Sutra. Find out how in this book. I know everybody has his or her way of having sex. However, if you stick to only one sexual move, how would you know what pleases you more. In this book, I'd also give you a detailed description of how to have nothing less than 10 different sexual positions.

Kama Sutra is one of the most fantastic books written about sexuality. When you have learned ultimately all you need to know about it, you will notice a turn around in your sexual like. I guarantee you! Remember when I told you it is possible to make your woman have an orgasm faster than she used to; with the right gameplay and technique, she'd have multiple orgasms. You also would have the best orgasm you've never had in your life.

Kama Sutra is very beneficial in all aspects. And this book would enlighten you on all you need to know about Kama Sutra. When you're done reading this book, you can be sure that your partner would love you more. You'd notice your partner wants to be around you always and they always feel turned on by you. All these secrets are in this book, so keep reading.

Also, I perceive you are having a weird feeling about the whole idea of Kama Sutra and all. You may probably be thinking right now that you love all that you've been hearing, but you don't seem to know how to bring the whole game changer to your life and the bedroom.

Well, you can talk to your partner about it, they might understand. But if you feel talking to your partner about Kama Sutra is out of the picture, don't worry, there are other ways you can maneuver it into your relationships. So, don't worry, in this book, I'd also teach you how to bring Kama Sutra into your life.

When you start applying Kama Sutra in your relationship, the result is fantastic. So, don't think about it too much. Our past is past, and there's nothing you can do about our past. So, don't live in the past. The future isn't here yet, but we dream of how we want it, despite that don't live in them. Instead of living in the past or present, live in the present and what you do currently. So, take a bold step today and learn more about the Kama Sutra.

Enjoy!

Chapter 1: What Is Kama Sutra?

When you hear the word Kama Sutra, what comes to your mind? Now, if sex comes to your mind, then you're on track. Kama Sutra is an ancient Sanskrit Indian text written on emotional fulfillment, eroticism, and sexuality in life. You shouldn't think of Kama Sutra as a manual on sexual positions, because it is not. Although Kama Sutra talks about sex position, but it isn't a manual, like the manual you get for your TV. You know your TV manual tells you to press the on button to switch the TV on, the Kama Sutra doesn't work that way. Instead see the Kama Sutra as a guide. Kama Sutra as a whole was written as a guide to the nature of love, maintaining one's love life, finding a life partner, and the art of living. Kama Sutra also talks about other aspects as it relates to pleasure-oriented faculties in our lives.

So, it would be wrong of you to expect to read the Kama Sutra and expect it to work like 1 + 1 = 2. It doesn't work that way. Kama Sutra is an art, and to fully enjoy the pleasures thereof; you need to understand the art as a whole. And when you know the technique, you'd know how to apply it as it affects you in your life. What works for me in my bedroom might be different from what works for John Doe. What makes girls attracted to me might be different from what makes girls attracted to you. So, the Kama Sutra is a guide that shows you how to use what you have to your advantage.

Kama Sutra is one of the oldest Hindu text about erotic love that has survived till date. It is a literary text with concise aphoristic verses that have survived even into the modern era with different commentaries and expositions. The Kama Sutra is a mix or Anustubh-meter and prose verses. One thing about the text I love so much is that it acknowledges the Hindu concept of Purusharthas (righteousness, prosperity, love, and spiritual values). It also lists desire, emotional, and sexual fulfillment as one the proper goal in life.

Basically speaking, Kama Sutra talks about a whole lot of things that can benefit our lives. But before we dive deeper into the benefits of Kama sutra, let us do a little background check on Kama sutra.

Background of Kama Sutra

The Hindu tradition holds the concept of Purusharthas as vitality for human sustenance. Now, the Purusharthas is divided into four main goals as already stated above. Dharma signifies righteousness, Artha signifies prosperity, Kama signifies love with or without sexual connotations, and Moksha signifies spiritual values. These four outlines are necessary for any human being to live a fulfilling and happy life.

Other lingual like Dharmasastra, Kamasastras, Arthasastras, and Mokshasastras genre have all done the same study on sexuality. As at the time they were making their studies, they saved their texts in palm leaves. Funny enough, most of these palm leaves has survived many years.

Kama sutra itself belongs to the Kamasastra genre of texts. Another example of Sanskrit text on emotions and sexuality is the Anangaranga, Ratirahasya, Panchasayaka, Nagarasarvasva, and Kandarpachudamani.

Professor Laura Desmond, is an anthropologist, and professor of Religious Studies. He claims that one of the defining objects of Indian Kamasastra literature is the harmonious sensory experience from a good relationship between yourself and the world. When you can understand this fully, you would be able to enhance your sensory capabilities in a way that it affects and can be affected by the world. Kama sutra has profited many such that it has been able to survive so many years.

Basically speaking on the Kama Sutra, it has survived via many versions throughout the Indian subcontinent. In an attempt to get the right translation of the Sanskrit Kama text in Anangaranga (a lingual widely translated by the Hindus in regional languages like Marathi), the associates of the British Orientalist Richard Burton came in contact with a part of the Kama sutra. In no time, the Brits had an intense love for the little portion of the sutra they had. They even commissioned the Sanskrit scholar Bhagvanlal Indraji to locate the complete Kama sutra, and translate the manuscript.

Indrajit did as commissioned, locating different variants of the manuscripts from libraries and temples of Varanasi, Jaipur, and Kolkata. Richard Burton then published a translated English edition of the manuscript, although it was not a critical edition of the Kama Sutra Sanskrit.

According to S.C. Upadhyaya, there were issues with Richard Burton published manuscripts that has survived. The text likely went through a lot of revisions over time. This was, however, confirmed by other 1st millennium CE Hindu texts on the Kama. There was mention and cite in the Kama Sutra and some quotations that credited the Kama Sutra by some historical authors, and were not found in his text of Kama Sutra that survived.

However, Vatsyayana, an ancient Indian philosopher is the first author to translate the Sanskrit text into English originally. He mainly discusses the Kama text based on its relationship with Artha and Dharma. However, he made some mentions of the fourth aim of life in some of the verses.

All being said, enough of the names and languages, let's proceed forward a little bit. At least by now, you already know the basics of the Sanskrit Kama, as well as the major for aims in life the Kama Sutra is all about.

What does Kama Sutra talk about?

Having said all that about the history and built a solid foundation of where Kama Sutra came from, let's go deeper. Now, let me enlighten you a bit on what the book talks about. In Vatsyayana's Kama Sutra, there were 1250 verses and 36 chapters in 64 sections, and it was infused in 7 books.

Kama Sutra makes use of a combination of prose and poetry to narrate the dramatic fiction of two characters, Nayika (Woman) and Nayaka (Man). These characters were aided by other characters like Vita (Pander), Pitamarda (Libertine), and Vidushaka (Jester). What is doing by these characters can be subdivided into five main acts. Allow me to break down the happenings below.

Flirting and Courtship

A couple of acts in the text includes several events and happenings where the subjects were flirting, which resonates in the modern era today. For instance, there was a place that suggests that if a man, not just any man, a young man, to be precise, seeks to attract a woman, he should hold a party. And at the party, he should invite guests to recite poetry. In the modern-day, we can replace poetry with something else. Perhaps a Dj, or a rapper, or a singer would suffice for a perfect replacement of the poet.

Another example is a text from Kama Sutra that suggests a boy and a girl should play together, probably go swimming in the river. Then the boy should dive into the water away from the girl he likes. The boy should then swim under the water to her, then surprise her by touching her gently from her legs upwards, then dive in again and swim away from her. In the modern era, you can still try this, and it works perfectly every single time. Even if you are at the beach, river, swimming pool, it all works perfectly well with this tip.

Book 3 of Kama Sutra talks mainly in the art of courtship with the aims of marriage. At the opening verse of book 3, there is a declaration that marriage should be a conducive means of purely natural love between partners. The first three chapters of the book talks about how a man needs to find the right bride. And the fourth chapter is about how a woman can get the man she desires.

Intimacy and Foreplay

Vatsyayana's Kama Sutra also describes foreplay and intimacy in many forms before and during sex. In this part, that is where we'd talk about foreplay like the embrace. In Kama Sutra, embrace (Alingana) is discussed in eight forms. These eight forms of Alingana includes Sphrishtaka, Viddhaka, Udghrishtaka, Piditaka, Lataveshtitaka, Vrikshadhirudha, Tilatandula, and Kshiranira. In embrace text from Kama Sutra, the first four are grouped into what is called expressive mutual love, which is rather non-sexual. The other four are grouped into increased pleasure during foreplay and during sexual intimacy.

And for the intimacy part of the Kama text involves kissing (Chumabanas). The text suggests that there are twenty-six different types of kisses. The types of kisses range from those kiss that shows affection to those that shows respect, and then during foreplay and sex. Vatsyayana also made mention of the different kissing practices in different parts of ancient India. Other forms of intimacy and foreplay include, holding, and embraces, rubbing, and mutual massage. Intimacy and foreplay also include biting and pinching, hands to stimulate, and using fingers, three styles of French kissing, and different styles of cunnilingus and fellatio.

Adultery

You'd probably wondering what the Kama Sutra says about adultery, right? Well, there are about 16 verses in the Sutra that talks about the reasons why a man is free to seduce a married woman. Vatsyayana also mentions several types of urban girls who are unmarried virgins, some were married but abandoned by husbands, and others were windows looking to remarry and courtesans.

Vatsyayana also encouraged young ones to learn how to earn a living. He further continued that because their young age is for pleasure, and as the years pass, they should concentrate on living virtuously and hope to escape the circle of rebirth. Kama Sutra teaches a man adulterous sexual affairs in a way that it allows a woman to assist him such that it works against his enemies and also facilitates his successes.

In the Sutra, there are citations which explain the signs and reasons why a woman wants to go into an adulterous relationship. It also explains the reasons why she does not want to commit adultery. The Kama Sutra teaches the strategies on how to engage in an adulterous relationship. However, it concluded the chapter on sexual affairs, stating that it is not advisable for anyone to go into an adulterous relationship. The Sutra claims that adultery benefits only one side of the marriage and not the two sides, thereby leaving the other hurting. Moreover, adultery goes against Artha and Dharma.

Caste, Class

When talking about uniqueness, Kama Sutra is a unique sociological and cultural milieu of ancient India. There is a near-total disregard for caste (jati) and class (varna) in Kama Sutra. The human relationship as it pertains to different sexual type are not segregated either was it repressed by caste or gender. In the pages of Kama Sutra, the lovers are not high class, neither were they, low class, either, they were at least rather rich enough to dress and wear proper clothing. The characters also pursuit after social leisure activities, and buy surprise gifts for their lovers.

The only rare mention of caste (i.e., High class) was in a text when a man was finding his legal wife and also advice about stories on how to seduce a woman especially other virgins of the same jati (castes). Generally, the text talks about sexuality between a man and woman across different caste and class both in rural and urban settings.

Same-sex, Group-sex Relationships

Lastly, Kama text also talks about homosexual relationships, such as oral sex between two women, as well as between two men. Lesbian relationships are covered mainly in chapter 5 and 8 of Vastyaayana's Kama Sutra. Same-sex relationships were explained in Kama Sutra through the notion of the third sexuality (Tritiya Prakriti).

The text discusses that there are two sorts of third nature. The first third nature is when a man behaves or thinks he's a woman. The second notion is when a woman behaves of think she's a man. There is a long conservative text in the Sutra that talks about a man dressed in a woman's apparel having fellatio with another man. There are also places where a two-woman losing their virginity with each other using their fingers, as well as sex toys and oral sex.

In this book, we'd be talking about everything Kama Sutra. We'd be featuring how to kiss and caress your partner, massage, foreplay, as well as different ways of making love. So, sit back and relax as we take you on an adventure.

Chapter 2: How can I Apply this to my Life in the Modern Day

It is no surprise if you have this question in your mind. The Kama Sutra is an ancient book. And as we'd have it, times have changed. But has our sexual desires as humans evolved? Well, the short, simple answer to that is no. It's pretty much the same. And if you'd ask me what I feel, well, I think the ancient guys had their sexual life figured out than we do. So, if you want to know how to apply Kama Sutra to your life in the modern world, stick around.

No matter how time changes, our want for a loving, and desirable and compassionate partner that we can connect with would never change. In the Hindu tradition where Kama Sutra sprang out from, saw the human body as a vehicle that is used to express spirituality and not as the West see it for many centuries as a sinful thing. Sex is famed as a sacrament and the joy of having sex. The wall carving and erotic status in many Hindu temples is an indication of the celebration of sex.

The bottom line is that sex should not be worshipped, as many people do in the modern world. To truly enjoy sex to the fullest, you need to take it from the grass root, and then build it up to something great. Seeing a lady in a bar, and you walk up to her to buy her a drink, and after 5 minutes of conversation, you guys are already in a room having sex. And in 10 minutes you are done – that isn't sex. What you guys are indulging in, is called FUCKING! Fucking is different from having sex or making love.

Fucking is when all you guys care about is the penis and the vagina. When all other factors is equal to zero, when you care more about you having an orgasm, then that is fucking. Fucking can be somewhat greedy, because all you care about is yourself, and your pleasure. But on the other hand, real sex takes more than just the penis and vagina to have. To have real sex, it doesn't start with clothes going off.

Real sex takes time; it builds up; it grows, and all the little things you do before and during sex, is what makes it real sex. There are also lots of emotions flying everywhere when having real sex; it's more like your partner is in your head, stimulating all the right places. It's more like when you're being touched right at that spot you want every single time.

Many people have fucked, but very few have had real sex. But don't worry, because today, we're going to be talking about everything you need to know about having that deep connection. Now to introduce Kama Sutra and start having real sex in this modern world, there are some few steps you need to take. So, without any further ado, let's get right into the details.

Preparing the Body

The first and most crucial part about introducing the Kama to the bedroom is by first preparing the body. Preparing the body can be equated with cleanliness. It starts with you as an individual. If you want to bring this whole Kama story into reality in your life in a modern-day, then you need to take your cleanliness seriously.

As a man or as a woman, when you wake up in the morning, brush your teeth, use the toilet, take your bath. It doesn't matter if you're married or single; it applies to everyone. Preparing the body should be done individually. But if you feel you have a deeper connection with your partner and you don't mind doing it together, kudos to that.

As a man always try to do a little work out in the morning so that your body would feel fit. If possible, a walk or jog around the block would suffice. And if you can do more exercise to have a somewhat fit or athletic physique that would equally work. Before you go out for the workout, (if you're jogging) make sure you brush your teeth. Also, make sure you don't wear a sweaty clothes (meaning make sure you don't have a bad body odor). The reason why you should care is that you never know who you might run into, so it's better if you're always prepared.

As a woman, you should also do the same. You should also do a little workout, so you don't lose your body shape. Brush your teeth regularly and take your bath regularly. Don't always wait till you have a smelling body odor oozing out before your shower. As a man or a woman, when preparing your body, there are two essential things you need always to do either together or alone.

Perfuming the Breath

An odor from any part of the body dampens sexual passion. No matter how high in the sexual spirit, you think you may feel, a big mood-killer is an odor. And what is even worse is when you combine body odor with bad breath that alone would kill the mood stone dead. The Kama text highly recommends that as a person, you should improve on your breath for better sexual experience. Luckily for you, there are a couple of breath freshener in the market you can get. In Vatsyayana's Kama Sutra, he suggested betel leaves, and you'd agree with me that most of the breath freshener out there today are better. So, this should be to your advantage in being in the modern-day.

A lot of people who are suffering from bad breath today don't even know they have bad breath. And most times, because their partner does not want to sound offensive or rude, they don't mention it, which usually causes a lot of problems. So, feel free to ask your partner to be honest with you if you have bad breath. At least your partner would feel more comfortable disclosing whether you have bad breath or not if you requested him or her to tell you. However, in a case where the mouth odor is rather intense, you should seek medical advice rather than disguising the problem with mouth freshener.

Bathing Together

Bathing together is another way of preparing the body to bring Kama teachings into the bedroom in a modern world. When you and your partner take a shower together or share a bathtub, it sets the mood right. It takes away the grime of the day, and it also creates an atmosphere for love. The two of you can also add a little foreplay to the picture. For whatever makes you feel comfortable. Don't be too pushy; likewise, don't restrict yourself to just bathing alone.

Always pay attention to your partner's body languages. Know when they want more of you, and when they want their space. If they want their space, it means you haven't quite set the mood right, and you need to try another approach. The takeaway message is that you make sure you do what makes you both comfortable and don't force yourself to enjoy the moment. True lovemaking comes naturally.

The Erogenous Zones

Another approach from the Kama teachings that can be brought to the bedroom in a modern-day is the erogenous zones. The erogenous zones or better still the pleasure zones are those parts of the body that turns your partner on, sets them in the mood. It is said that the brain is the most potent sexual organ, which is very accurate. The brain is one of the most important parts of sex, and engaging it while making love is very vital as well. Lovemaking without the imagination free play is more like a soulless mechanical activity; better still we call it fucking.

As good lovers, it's essential to have an imaginative and sensitive appreciation of those parts of each other's body that are referred to as erogenous zones. No sexually active person would deny the fact that the genitals are the primary erogenous zones. However, other erogenous zones needs to be tapped in other to have the potential erotic and extreme joy of making love. For example, the brain, and the skin are two more primary erogenous zones that shouldn't be left out of the picture.

Concentrating on just the primary erogenous zones of the body and leaving out the myriads of other erogenous zones is like eating part of a well-balanced diet and then leaving the remaining part out. Kama Sutra speaks widely on the topic of pleasure zones and that they should be exploited. Of kissing, for instance, Kama text suggested some places that should be kissed, like the lips, in the mouth, the cheeks, throats, forehead, and so on.

There are also other pleasure zones like the breasts, the nipples, buttocks, earlobes, feet, and the list goes on and on. Some people are turned on by having their calves touched and inside their arm. And for others, it could be anywhere on their skin. Let me enlighten you on these pleasure zones.

Lips and Throats

To some people, a kiss on the lips or at the throat is what sets them in the mood. So a spine-tingling aroused, a light kiss or lick around the throat would suffice. You could also lightly touch the throat as well. Many people have successfully used these erogenous zones to seduce a lot of women. Now you know the drill, feel free to try it out as it works perfectly fine in a modern world.

Best Foot Forward

The best foot forward talks about everything you need to know about the foot, and it's erogenous zones. There are reflex connections in the feet as well as the rest of the body. When these reflex connections are stimulated, we feel goose pimples all over our body (you should be able to relate with this). The sensation flows from the limbs to the rest of the body, especially the head. Some people only relate to feet and sex to foot fetishism. However, the pleasures of the feet go way deeper. Here are some erogenous zones on the feet that sets the right mood.

Ankles and calves: You can have some surprising sensual feelings by simple stimulating some parts of the ankles, toes, and calves. While grooming the body for sex, you can occasionally slide your hands around your partner's body and locate these points. You can also combine it with a soft, gentle kiss on their lips to even set the mood higher up.

Thighs: The tights are also very sensitive parts for both male and female. It's muscular and soft. So, a lot of feelings goes on around there. You can also slide your hand in the sensitive inner thigh of your partner. You could even slide it further down, and go closer to the genitals, and play around it. You could also place a kiss on the thigh or lick around it with your tongue for real erotic pleasure.

Buttocks: buttocks is one of the most popular erogenous zones. The buttocks are richly enriched with nerve cell, so every squeeze and spanking goes a long way. It all depends on what you're partner prefers. Use the body language of your partner to decide.

Sensual Skin

The skin is the largest organ we have, as it is one of the erogenous zones; it should be one of the most exploited. The skin is sensitive to the lightest touch and the smallest change to temperature and pressure. There are also over 1500 sensory receptors in the skin, so yes it very touch sensitive. Although the sensual feeling from the skin depends on the part or erogenous zone touched.

The Breasts: The woman's breast has a significant role it plays in sexual attraction. It doesn't only attracts the man but it also an undeniable pleasure zone for the woman, and the man. The nipple areas are surrounded by areolae, which are highly sensitive to touch. So, when you rub her nipples softly, it gets to her head. At times when you combine it with a little sucking, it gets deep into her head, which is characterized by her closing her eyes to enjoy the full pleasure thereof. At times while squeezing her nipples and breasts, she could bite her lips and stare intensely at the man to give him a devout, please.

The Buttocks: a lot of men find a woman's buttock very attractive. It doesn't end there because the buttock is also a sensitive, sensual part of the skin. The buttocks can be a pleasure house and an attractor. It can be mutually stimulating when a man squeezes, and lightly slaps the buttocks. He could also kiss and bite the buttocks gently. The woman, on the other hand, can also indulge in the act and find it as enjoyable too. For a slight variation in the ways you want to stimulate the buttocks, you can try using light strokes combined with loses and gentle but firm squeezes and kneading.

Anal sensitivity: lastly, there is anal sensitivity. For many who haven't tried anal sex before, you might want to consider trying it. Anal sex might be somewhat painful at first, but it's very pleasurable. For stimulating the anal, you could start with your fingers. Imagine a clock face on your partner's anus, and 12 o'clock hand being the part that points to the tentacles or the vagina. Using that clockface imagination of your partner's anus, locate 2 o' clock, and 10 o' clock as they are the most sensitive points.

Creating the Mood

The same way it is important to prepare the body, as well as it is to locate the erogenous zones, it is equally important to create the right mood. In creating the right mood, there are a couple of things you can use to create the right atmosphere which would give room for the right mood to set in. One of the first suggestion is to make sure that if the weather is hot, make the room refreshingly cool. Also in cold weather, make the room warm enough, but don't make it stuffy. Having background music also helps to create the right mood. However, the music shouldn't be too raucous or agitated, but something conducive and tender, but not too soporific so you don't feel sleepy. Despite the way loving making is done in the modern world in the Kama text things are a bit different, you'd agree with me that by following the Kama text, you'd do better. Here are some quick tips on what you can use to create the right mood.

Flowers

Flowers has been one of everyone's favorite things when making love. Flower is a perfect way of connecting us to that inner feeling we have inside. When you want to create the perfect environment in your room for lovemaking, sprinkles fresh fragrant flowers like roses in the room. You can use the roses to decorate and perfume your room so that when you both step into the room, the whole atmosphere just seems perfect and out of this world. Everything quickly falls into place when the flowers are red.

Soft Light

Another idea you should engage in is making use of soft light. The light shouldn't be too dull so that you can still see each other. Likewise, the light shouldn't be too bright, so the atmosphere doesn't seem too busy. You could set gently flickering glow of candlelight in your room as they are more romantic than electric light. For safety reasons, keep candles away from curtains bedding or any flammable materials in the room. You can swap make use of scented candles as they lit the room and equally perfume it as well. Candles are generally preferred because they create a kind of soft and seductive light.

Scenting the Room

Scenting the room is equally important when trying to create the right mood. Anything that makes the nose work has an indirect connection with the brain. Having a nice scenting room is a perfect way to seduce any woman. You can also make use of seductive scented like invents scented crystals, or heated essential oil. Whichever type of scent you decide to use, all works perfectly.

Champagne and Silk

Having a bottle of well-chilled vintage champagne with seductive silk lingerie or nightmare goes a long way in making the environment even more perfect. For a romantic evening, whether at a hotel or home, be sure to indulge in using silk and champagne.

Perfuming the Skin

I have spoken about this point before, and I don't want to overemphasize on it, as you also ready know what you need to do. Have a nice body fragrance. When you have your bath, use a delicately scented bathing oil to perfume your skin. And if you're more of a shower kind of person, use a scented shower gel. Always make sure you gave a fresh body fragrance.

Oil and Lotions

To make your foreplay even more seductive, engage in using oils and lotions. Using scented massage oil and lotion on each other's skin is even more pleasurable. There are different ways in which you can give each other a sensual massage; we would talk more about it later in this book.

Chapter 3: How to Introduce Kama Sutra to the Bedroom in Today's World

In this chapter of the book, we'd be talking about how to introduce Kama sutra to the bedroom in today's world. I would be using teachings from the Kama sutra to explain how it still applies to our sexual lives even in the modern world.

There is this particular teaching from the Kama text that particularly caught my attention, and I would be sharing it with you. It talks about touching and caressing. When you look deep into touching and caressing, although it's still a part of foreplay, there is more to it than meets the eye. What interested me the most is that the best strategy to use to introduce Kama teachings to the bedroom in a modern world is by using the lessons of touching and caressing from Kama Sutra.

Touching and caressing is a vast topic to cover. You can even use a part of touching and caressing to connect with your partner deeply. We'd cover this part of touching and caressing in the next chapter. But in this chapter, we'd focus on the part of touching and caressing you can use to introduce Kama teachings to the bedroom in a modern world.

There are a couple of things for you to learn from this text. So, I suggest you get your learning mind up and ready to receive a newly added knowledge to get you on track. So, let's get right into it.

What is touching and caressing?

Touching and caressing is an act of physically stimulating your partner's erogenous zones for pleasurable sensual moments. Touching and caressing is a form of foreplay generally encouraged to be done before sex and during sex. There are different types of touching and caressing, and each comes with its advantages over the other.

When you touch a particular part of your partner's body, and it feels very sensual, it doesn't mean you're to only concentrate on only that part. A combination of different stimulation of the various erogenous zones is what leads to great lovemaking.

Under touching and caressing from the Kama teachings, there are five major lessons I will be covering in this book. These lessons include embracing, mutual grooming, sensual massage, scratching, and hair play. These different lessons are what we are going to use to explain this chapter and the next. In other words, you can use the teaching from touching and caressing to introduce the Kama into the bedroom and also profoundly connect with your partner. In this chapter, we would be talking mainly on embracing and mutual grooming.

Embracing

Embracing from the Kama Sutra is divided into up to eight different kinds. Of the eight types of embracing, they are divided into two groups. The first group includes four kinds of embrace which talk about different embracing that indicates the mutual love between a man and a woman coming together. The first group comprises embracing such as the touching embrace, the rubbing embrace, the piercing embrace, as well as the pressing embrace.

This second group of embrace also includes four types of embrace that involves a somewhat more intimate kind of embrace. This group of embrace consists of the mixture of sesame seed with rice embrace (Tila Tandulaka), climbing a tree embrace (Vrikshadhirudhaka), the twinning of a creeper (Jataveshtitaka), and the milk and water embrace (Kshiraniraka).

Apart from these significant types of embrace, you can quickly learn and use in the bedroom; the Vatsyayana Kama also talks about four different ways you can embrace simple members of the body. These include simple members of the body like the breasts, thighs, the forehead, and the middle part of the body (Jaghana). Having a full understanding of how the embrace works would give you a complete insight into how to introduce the Kama into the bedroom in a modern-day. So, without further ado, let's dive into the details of how this embrace works.

1. The First Group of Embrace

In this group of embrace, we would be talking about a little bit, not too intense way to embrace your partner. This types of embrace do not have too much sensual feeling in it, and you can easily practice it even when you do not want to have sex. And on the topic of embrace, here is takeaway advice, using a couple of embraces mixed with other foreplay is a perfect way to start lovemaking. All you need to take note of are your partner's soft spots. Triggers those sweet spots and combine it with the right embrace and you'd find everything falling into place.

This group of embrace is straightforward, and sometimes can even be practiced in public places. There isn't really much to this group of embrace. Also, a lot of people practice most of the embrace in this group without even knowing it belongs to this group. What I am trying to say is that it is the most common type of embrace out there. The benefits of this embrace is that it is straightforward and can be used to lure your partner easily. So, when you really want to introduce the Kama into the bedroom, be sure to start with any one of the embraces in this group.

1) The Touching Embrace

The touching embrace is a type of embrace whereby the man stands in front of the women and their body touches. This embrace is all about making sure your bodies touch; you feel the warmth of your partner's body. Your bodies should also touch in a way that you feel the texture of your partner in a way that you can tell how soft or hard your partner's body is.

This type of embrace can be a playful way of showing erotic affection to your partner. Take, for instance, when you step into the room, and your partner walks up to you with arms wide open. And the man shoves you into his arms. And you as the woman falls into his arms and find that comfort spot, where you can feel his body warmth, and soft but a bit rigid muscles. And then you dim your eyes a bit with a little smile on your face. That scenario is a perfect example of a touching embrace. Note that the key point of this embrace is the bodies coming in contact.

2) The Rubbing Embrace

The rubbing embrace, on the other hand, is a type of embrace where two partners rub their bodies together. For instance, imagine two lovers walking down a dark street, or a public place like a resort, or somewhere a bit lonely. When these two lovers in this scenario rub their bodies against each other as they walk is called the rubbing embrace. This type of embrace is best done when you are in public or walking together. This type of embrace is mainly common among the younger ones when walking together with their arms tightly around their partner's waist.

Nonetheless, you can perfectly practice this embrace even in the house. In the kitchen, for example, when you're both fixing a meal, perhaps you want to go to the other side of the kitchen, you can pass by your partner, and rub your body against theirs with a big smile on your face. There are different ways you can apply the rub embrace; the main point here is to rub your body against each other. I said rub, not hold or press, that the main difference, the rubbing part.

3) The Pressing Embrace

The pressing embrace is one of my favorite types of embrace. This type of embrace is a lot more sensual, with a whole lot of emotions attached to it. This type of embrace is very similar to the touching embrace, but the main difference between the two is that the touch embraces the main objective is to make sure there is contact. But for the pressing embrace, the main objective is to make sure that there isn't just contact, but the contact is deep and forcibly against your partner's body.

In this type of embrace, the woman can even feel the man's heart beating because of how tight the body would be pressed against each other. This embrace is mostly given when a party misses the other, and they want to get all they have missed in a big hug. This type of embrace is very common among young lovers as they get pinned to the wall or pillar by their lover. Being pinned to the wall or pillar by a lover is a type of embrace only a few people would object to.

4) The Piercing Embrace

Lastly, the piercing embrace is a type of embrace that is even more sensual than the pressing embrace. If you try to figure out what this embrace means from the name would clearly misdirect you as the word piercing used is merely a figure of speech and not a literal description. What the piercing embrace is all about is when a woman brushes her breast against her man as she bends.

To perform this embrace, let's do a little bit of imagination. Imagine a man sitting or standing whichever one you prefer, then imagine a woman in front of him and his hands around her waist. Now that you have that picture in your mind, that perfect, now imagine the woman bending backwards as though she wants to pick something from the floor. She doesn't need to bed too backward; the aim is to expose her breast.

Now, as the breasts are exposed, the man grips her even closer to his bosom, and the embrace is complete as he feels the warmth and softness of her breast. This type of embrace is very sensual and has a lot of emotion attached to it.

2. The Second Group of Embrace

This group of embrace is a combination of embracing and lovemaking. This group of embrace is very sensual and very stimulating. This type of embrace can also be adopted during the congress or lovemaking. Don't worry yourself too much about the names of each of the embrace; I know they sound a bit off. But the main thing you should focus your mind on is understanding how the embrace works. Here are the four types of embrace in this group.

1) The Milk and Water Embrace

If you are still new into the whole love game, and you and you're very much into each other, then this type of embrace is perfect for you. Although this type of embrace and lovemaking might be a bit painful, because you and your partner are too much in love with each other, you wouldn't be thinking of any hurt or pain.

To perform this embrace, imagine a man in a seated position on a chair or on the bed and the woman on his lap. As the man sits with a full-blown penis, the woman comes and sits on it as she embraces him with her hands around his back, and the man's hand around her back as well. Lovemaking would be a lot slower, but it would be very passionate. Lovers would try these types of embrace and lovemaking eventually lose themselves to each other in their physical relationship.

2) Climbing a Tree Embrace

Climbing a tree embrace is a pretty simple embrace to perform. In this embrace, the woman places one of her feet on the foot of her lover, and the other foot is placed on one of his thighs. One of her arms also goes round to his back, and the other one stays on his shoulder. She could also talk dirty like how she would want the make to fuck her or so whatever turns the man on. Then she should try as though she is making an attempt to climb his for a kiss.

As her leg is on one of the man's thighs, he should go for the penetrations. Also, note that this type of lovemaking might also be somewhat painful. But with the amount of love as well as other factors between lovers, make them ignores this pain.

3) The Mixture of Sesame Seed with Rice Embrace

The mixture of sesame (Sesamum) seen with rice embrace is a type of embrace lover do while lying down on the bed. In this embrace, the lovers lie on the bed and embrace each other closely, with arms and thighs of one of the lovers encircled by the arms and thighs of the other lover. In that position, they rub their thighs and arms against each other while they make love as it were like the mixture of sesamum seed with rice.

From the name of this embrace, the sesame seed with rice signifies the thighs and the arms of the lovers, and the mixture signifies them rubbing together. The main aim of this embrace is to have maximum skin-to-skin contact.

4) The Twining of a Creeper Embrace

Lastly, we would be looking at this type of embrace in this group. Kama Sutra describes this embrace as when a woman clings to her man as a creeper twines around a tree. The man then bends his head down to as he reaches to kiss her. And then he makes a little sound like shh, as they embrace. And then the woman looks lovingly towards him and have a cute smile on her face.

In this embrace, as the man put your hands around her back as though you supporting her from falling back. And the woman holds the man's neck with one hand and leaned her head towards the man's shoulder. One of the woman's legs also goes to the side of the man's thigh as the man holds it with his second hand. Then the embrace is complete with that passionate look.

3. Embracing Simple Members of the Body

The main aim of embracing the simple members of the body is the arousal of the male desire. It includes embracing simple parts of the woman's body with the intention of causing arousal in the man's desire. There are four types of embracing simple members of the body. Although in the holy book of Kama, there are orders in which embrace should be followed; however, in a case where the wheel of love sets in, there are no motion and no order.

1) Embracing the Thighs

You may be wondering how embracing the thighs can help in introducing the Kama to the bedroom, well it is because it causes arousal. To perform this type of embrace is done when a lover presses forcibly one or both of the thighs against the partners own. In an attempt to bring the thighs together, you would feel your genitals touching each other, which would cause an increase in your desire and arousal. This type of embrace is sensual, and you should try it out. As your lover presses their body against yours, on full arousal, the lover can move naturally on to intercourse.

2) Embracing the Jaghana

Performing the Jaghana or middle part of the woman's body embrace is one type of embrace you should check out. To perform this embrace, the man presses her Jaghana against your own and mount on her to either bite, scratch with the finger or nail, strike softly, kiss, or play with her hair softly. The Jaghana, according to Kama Sutra, is the area between the thighs and the navel. Clearly, with this type of embrace, congress preludes.

During the congress, as you penetrate her vagina and feel that warm, and wet sensation, you can follow it by sliding your pelvis against her combining it with a circular up and down movement for optimal joy. However, in this modern-day, a lot of lovers often give up on the biting, kissing, and scratching part of this ritual. Although it is not bad if you want to take those parts of the ritual off, the main aim of the embrace is to do what makes you feel comfortable the most.

3) Embracing the Forehead

We can also call this embracing affectionate nuzzling. To perform this embrace with your partner, reach out to your lover and touch their mouth, eyes, forehead with your own. This times of embrace can be used to build up intimacy quickly, confidence with your partner, as well as also enhance arousal. Feel free to engage in this embrace and see where it leads you and your lover.

4) Embracing the Breasts

As a lover, you can also practice embracing the breast as a way to introduce the teachings from the Kama to the bedroom. To perform this embrace, as a man, place your chest or breast between the breasts of your lover. Then press your chest against your lover's breasts so that you can feel the warmth and softness of your lover's breast. An upper body contact like this embrace creates a nipple stimulation for you and your lover. In the end, you would have a higher chance of changing from the usual oral caresses.

Mutual Grooming

In many verses in the Kama Sutra, it was mentioned several times that cleanliness should not be omitted by lovers. Mutual grooming is when you and your lover participate in helping each other stay clean. Mutual grooming can also be seen as a way of preparing the body by lovers for lovemaking. This preparation of the body can include, bathing or showering together, shaving the man's face, washing, drying, and then brushing each other's hair and so on. You can do whatever makes you both feel comfortable.

There are different ways lovers can both mutually groom each other, but we would be focusing on two major ways you can groom each other. Mutual grooming is an indispensable ritual and is highly recommended for lovers. When couples focus their attention to each other's attraction, it can help elevate the anticipation of pleasure. Mutual grooming can help encourage feelings for trust, tenderness, caring, which will cause each partner to feel a kind of security towards the other. Engaging in any one of the following mutual grooming below can help break down inhibition in a new relationship and also help to reinforce the bonds of an established one.

1) Shaving his beard

From Kama teaching, it is recommended that a man should shave more often than every four days. This act can be somewhat challenging to keep up with.

Moreover, having grown beard and looking down at your woman to kiss her can be a mood killer. So, rather than you as a woman telling your man to shave, you can easily do the shaving for him. While you shave your man's beards, make sure you apply enough lather, this is to ensure that you end up with a smooth shave with no cuts.

Don't make the mistake of thinking shaving is for men only. Women also shave; they shave their armpits, legs, and some women shave their pubic hair. Some men prefer their woman to have a hairless pudendum as they find it very erotic. If a woman is also to shave her pubic hair, then she would need to shave it regularly. This is because new hair growth would quickly spring out after a shave, and the new growth would even be stronger and a bit sharp and spiky, which could irritate her lover's skin.

2) Shampooing her Hair

Shampooing your lover's hair is another way you can groom her. Some people even see shampooing her hair as a form of embrace. Although this isn't all that correct because shampooing isn't done during lovemaking, neither is it done for the same reasons embrace is being done. Even though shampooing is not an ideal embrace, it is very sensual grooming. Shampooing is a very intimate experience, especially when shared.

You would agree with me that, as lovers, you enjoy having a soapy bath, and drying each other's body before you go to bed. However, shampooing each other's hair can be a very affectionate moment of grooming, it might not lead to sex at the end of the day. However, it is a great way to start when you want to introduce Kama Sutra to the bedroom in a modern world.

Chapter 4: How to use this to Deeply Connect with my Partner

Now in this chapter, we would be talking about ways in which you can deeply connect with your partner. This chapter is somewhat a continuation of the lessons we were learning from the previous chapter (chapter 3). We were learning from the lessons of touching and caressing from Kama Sutra and how we can use it to bring Kama Sutra to the bedroom in the modern world. We also learned that under the teachings of touching and caressing, there are five different subdivisions. These subdivisions include embracing, mutual grooming, sensual massage, scratching, and hair play.

From the previous chapter, we also learned that embracing and mutual grooming and two subdivisions of touching and caressing that could be used to introduce Kama Sutra to the bedroom in the modern-day world. However, the remaining three branches of the touching and caressing can be used to connect with your partner deeply. In this chapter, we would be taking a closer look into the remaining subdivisions of touching and caressing and see that we can learn from it.

Sensual Massage

The message is one part of touching and caressing that should not be left out when talking about sex. As humans, we give a lot of references to touch as we tend to link it to sex one way or the other. Sometimes some people fear to touch themselves because of that fear of it being misunderstood. A massage is a form of touch, a very sensual touch that usually preludes congress most times between lovers. One of the most important reasons why people often require massage is to soothe away tension and tiredness.

A lot of lovers often skip or overlook the power of massage, and as such, they miss out on making the body more receptive and relaxed for making love in which they could use to connect with their partners deeply. Whether or not your intention of having a sensual massage session with your partner is to have sex, or not, the main aim of a sensual massage is to create a peaceful and comfortable setting for maximum relaxation. So, whenever you really want to connect with your lover deeply, a sensual massage always has a way of giving it to us.

To have a perfect sensual massage with your lover, a large bed with a firm mattress would do just fine. Or better still, you can place a sheet on the floor, which would be more suitable. Pillows should also be available which would serve as cushions for your lover's neck, back, and ankles. Also make the environment perfect by ensuring it is a bit warm, as well as softly lit. And for the best deepest connection between you and your lover, make sure there wouldn't be any interruption during the massage session. So, if your mobile phone or TV set would be a problem, be sure to do away with it for the time being, or better still switch it off.

There are also different massaging moves that you can use individually or combined with two or more of them. When you start the massage, build them into a full sequence whereby you start from the feet, and you work your way up to the head, and you go back and forth and around. There are different spots in which you are to massage to get the most out of the feeling. But before we look into that, let us first learn the basic massaging strokes. With the right massage stroke at the right spot, you would be a pro masseur or masseuse.

The Basic Massaging Strokes

There are different massage strokes you can use when massaging your lover. However, because of this lesson we are taking, we would be looking at five of the various basic massaging strokes you can use. Take note that whatever massaging stroke you decide to use, you should always try your best to keep your movement symmetrical, even and rhythmic. You should appropriately follow even stroke after the other.

If you want even to make things even more pleasurable, make use of suitable oil. There are different types of massaging oil in which we would also look into that briefly later in this chapter. When you apply the oil, always use the right amount of pressure that agrees with your partner's skin. Since massage is all about pleasure and not pain, be sure to always keep a check on the amount of pressure you are applying.

And at times during the massage, you may need to forgo your own pleasure or need and focus on your partner's enjoyment instead. By doing so, you will achieve your goal of being able to give your lover full pleasure. So, without further ado, here are the five different types of basic massaging strokes.

1) Tapotement and cupping

The tapotement and cupping massage stroke is a type of stroke that may involve you making use of both hands. Performing the tapotement massage stroke is more like your lover is lying down on the bed, and you do drumming with a light tapping action on your lover's body. On the other hand, to perform the cupping stroke, imagine your partner still lying down, you would pound his/her body with alternate hands sure that they form a cup with fingers together and your thumbs should be folded in.

2) Hacking

The hacking massage stroke is a type of stroke where you give your loves a series brisk chops with the side of your hand. This stroke is more like using your hand as in karate, but this time a lot gentler. When performing the hacking strokes on your lover's body, make sure you keep your fingers relaxed and not stiff.

3) Petrissage

For this massage stroke, move the balls of your thumb or fingers on your lover's body in a circular kind of motion. This stroke would help your lover soothe away any muscular tension that resides along the spine. Take note not to massage the spine itself as it could be very painful characterized with short sharp pains.

4) Kneading

If you are a fan of baking, if you knead bread dough of whatever type of dough, and you are good at it, then you would be equally as good in this type of massage stroke. To perform this stroke, use your hands to gently knead your lover's flesh in a curved, smooth, and regular movement.

5) Effleurage

The effleurage is a massage stroke that requires you to make use of your palm to glide on your lover's skin. As you glide on your lover's skin be sure to keep your body weight behind the movement, you do not want to put your weight forward, so it doesn't cause you to apply too much pressure. It would help when you make use of this massage stroke first and last on each area of the body your massage.

Using Massaging oil

If you ever decide to make use of messaging oil, be sure to pre-warm it before using it as it works best that way. So, when you pick the pick from its bottle or container, rub them for a few seconds between your hands to pre-warm the oil. When you want to start using the oil, apply it to a small area and attend to it before proceeding to another area rather than applying it to the whole body first before the massage.

After applying the oil to the intended area, follow it up with smooth yet firm strokes. Then when you are through with the massage, leave the oil on the skin to soak. On the other hand, you can wash the oil if you like by rubbing alcohol or gently wiping it off with a towel. However, because this has to be used cold, it might affect the effectiveness of the massage.

If you prefer, you can massage your partner with dry hands. Although massage with dry hands is also great, note that it would be smoother than when you make use of massage oil. There are different types of suitable oil with many gotten from nuts like coconut, and vegetable oils as well. There are also plain oils which are also great for massages such as almond, grapeseed, olive, and sunflower, which can be applied directly to the skin. A lot of people do make use of these plain oil as a base for perfumed essential oil, such as rose, jasmine, ylang-ylang, sandalwood, and patchouli. If you want to make a scented oil for a full massage session, then mix a dozen drop of essential oil with 30ml of base oil.

Different Areas on the Body to Massage

When talking about massage, there are specific areas on the body that should be massaged. On knowing these massaging spots, makes having a sensual massage a lot easier. This is because you would know exactly the right spot to go each time, and that would help you to connect with your partner deeply. There are up to six different areas on the body that should be massaged.

1) Shoulder and Head

A lot of people often when they massage the shoulders and head, they only go for the top of the head, but the action is very similar to that used when washing your partner's hair. However, this is not a grooming move, so it should be more sensual than what you have when grooming each other. The proper way to massage the shoulder and head is to first start by massaging your lover's front shoulder.

Work your way to the sides of your lover's neck as you keep massaging and then cheeks and the jaw. You should not also neglect the temples and forehead. While massaging, you can occasionally run your fingers lightly to the chin and around and over your lover's lips, nose and eyes. As you keep massaging, most of your lover's erogenous zones would be pleasantly sensitized.

2) Back and Spine

When working on massaging the back, make use of gently yet erotic pressure to work your way upward from your lover's buttocks. Try to keep your hands as wildly outspread and level with each other. Also, make your thumbs push inward along you lover's spine as you grind deeper on your partners back.

As you continue the massage in the warm and softly lit room on your lover, work your way up to the base of her/his neck and then out to the shoulders before you then bring your hands down slowly to the sides of her/his buttocks. If your loves being massage in this particular area, feel free to repeat it about ten times or more.

3) Feet and Legs

When you feel like getting the whole massaging spirit to the next level, then you can get to the feet and legs massage. Tell your lover to lie face-down as it would be easier to massage the calves and ankles that way. With your partner at a face-down position, you should sit close so that you avoid straining your back, that way you would not need to stretch forward or bend to reach your partner. Also, hold her leg steadily with one of your hands while you massage it with your other hand.

To start the massage, start by kneading, stretching, and bending each of the feet upward. Then you can proceed by softly rubbing the areas between your lover's feet. Next, run your palm firmly on the soles of the feet and then also rub it along the tops. In turn, raise each of your partner's legs and a few times, rotate each of them until it feels relaxed and loose. Then you can gradually move up the leg and as you do so, pay special attention to the calves, back, and ankles of the thighs and knees. When massaging the feet and legs, there are two types of strokes you can use, the downward leg strokes and the upwards leg strokes.

- *The Downward Leg Stroke*: this is a stroke where you draw you hand smoothly downwards from the ankle to the knee, and then you squeeze the muscle of the calf gently with your fingertips.

- *The Upward Leg Strokes*: this is a stroke where you use the same sort of action as when you were doing the downward stroke, but this time you are drawing your hand back up from the knee to the ankle.

4) Buttocks

For the buttocks massage, your partner would still need to lie face-down, and you would be sited right beside your partner. Then place your hand on your partner's buttocks to feel the texture of your buttocks as you move your hands in a decisive circular motion. Press the buttock firmly at first for your pleasure and his too. A lot of people enjoy doing a downward buttock stroke; you can try that as well, but, you decide what you and your partner enjoy doing most. After you can then increasingly lightly massage the buttocks until your hands are barely just brushing the skin. You can then continue with squeezing each of the buttocks, in turn, following it with kneading.

5) Arm and Chest

The arm and the chest are other areas of the body perfect for massaging. For optimal pleasure, your partner should lie down facing up for this massage to create a kind of deep connection between the two of you as you can have eye contact. Start this message from the front of the shoulders, and then work your way down to the chest area. You can further proceed to the arms by using a gentle kneading action and again working your way downward.

After that, you can then find your way to the thighs using a kind of circular movement of your hands. To make it easier, rotate your right hand clockwise, and your left hand counterclockwise. Then knead the groin and the thighs and slowly move towards the navel and pubic area. Use gentle pressure when you get to this area because it would be more pleasurable. Then gently pass over the rib too and trace the shape of the pectorals and the breasts with your fingertip as you massage them softly.

6) Upper Back

Lastly, massaging the upper back can help you build a very solid and deep connection with your partner. When you want to massage the upper back, focus more on the muscle between the base of the neck and the shoulder blades. From there, you can bring your hands back down as you follow it with massaging the sides with your fingertips. Reduce the pressure you are using and then knead the back of the neck and shoulders.

Scratching

It is common among lovers to often use their fingernails to scratch their body has an expression of passion. At times scratching could be used to represent reconciliation after you and your lover had a quarrel. During lovemaking, adding a little twist of scratching to the mix can help you create a deep connection with your partner. Although not everyone finds them pleasurable, so always be on the lookout for what pleases your partner.

The Kama Sutra made mention of marks of passion on a young woman's throat or breast as it is a way of telling the world she has a lover. Such marks have always been a thing of admiration right from the times of Vatsyayana and the Kama Sutra. Back in those days, even when a stranger sees a woman with markings of nails on her breast, the stranger would be filled with excitement, love, and respect for her. The same thing applies for men with nail markings on his body.

The Kama Sutra also made mention of scratches as being made by lovers as a reminder of the love they have for each other even when they are apart. So, anytime a lover looks in the mirror and sees the mark, he would be reminded of who puts it there. Or in a scenario where the love keeps feeling slightly uncomfortable itch or a little pain caused by scratch, would also serve as a conviction of the love they have.

Vatsyayana further made mention that wives should not be seen bearing such marks of passion on their body. Although it isn't that it is wrong for her to have one, she is free for her to bear them in private places hidden from everyone else. This is because when a married woman does such, it reduces her respect in public eyes. Vatsyayana further concludes that there is nothing that makes increases love as much as the effects of markings with the nails and biting. So, if leaving passion marks on your livers body is not based on cruelty or anger, then both of you would definitely find it to be fun from time to time.

There are different ways in which harmless passion marks can be used on both partners to express their feelings for each other at the height of excitement during or before intercourse. There are four main types of making this ritualized markings on your lover's body namely, with the back of your hand, with your fingers, with your fist, and with the palm of your hand. Knowing the right ritualized violence for you is dependent on how much violence you enjoy.

Hair Play

The Kama Sutra was very firm when it acknowledges the fascination of the woman's hair is to a man. Kama Sutra further recommends women to learn how to wash, perfume properly, and braid her hair. When a woman knows how to fond and praise her hair, it has the power to arouse feelings of desire in her partner. There are different forms in which lovers can play with hair to deeply connect with each other.

1) The Light Touch

When a woman has a long her, she could make it fall beguilingly over her lover's face and breast, then sensually bushes it against her partner's naked body. And if she is well graced with very long hair, she can enfold her hair on her lover's chest and shoulders. She should be on top in a way that she can sweep it over his entire body teasingly even on his penis so that it heightening his desire for her.

2) Revealing the Neck

A lustrous hair can be a very powerful aphrodisiac and can be inviting lovers to want to play with it and bury his hand in the hair. The texture and sheen of the hair is very attracted to your man. And when she lifts it too reveals a delicate and soft neck, and the joy even gets better.

3) Tactile Pleasure

As a couple, if you want a more intimate relationship that would allow you both to deeply connect with each other as you like, then you need to engage in a loving touch. Running your hand through your lover's hair and plays with the hair would increase the tactile pleasure for both of them.

Chapter 5: Kissing and Mouthplay in the Bedroom in Today's World

So far, so good, we have learned a lot from the Kama Sutra and how we can apply them to our lives. But now, let's talk about something a little different. Did you know kissing and mouth play, in general, can bring lots of passion to your relationship? A relationship without passion can be a rough one. So I would rather prefer you take advantage of anything that can bring passion to your relationship purely.

Kissing involves the use of your mouth, which is one of the most sensitive parts of the body. You could use your lips or tongue to lick, suck, kiss, and nibble or nozzle areas on your partner's body. Kissing is even art of its own you and your partner can use every day. And Kama Sutra recognizes the benefits of kissing and its different forms. The intensity of the way you kiss your partner has a role it plays on expressing your feelings to your partner. The intensity of a kiss uses a combination of three senses - smell, taste, and touch — each of these parts of the body produces a strong emotional response from your partner. Kissing ranges from fleeting contact to deep penetration with your tongue and so on. Let's dive into it a little bit more.

Types of kissing

There are different types of kissing teachings from the Kama Sutra we would be featuring. You can learn from them and apply then to express a lifting in your relationship. Here are the different types of kissing.

The Bent Kiss

Why not kiss your lover naturally today with this bent kiss. With your head angled slightly on one side which will allow you to get a maximum lip contact. You can even have a deep tongue penetration with this type of kiss, which is very sensual.

To perform this type of kiss, gently approach your partner and draw it very slowly as you head tilt to one side. You can pick any side you like - left or right. As you go for the kiss, take it slowly, let the lips touch first then after the full contact you then open your lips and play around with it before going for the deep penetration. You can also place your hand at the back of your partners head as you rub it gently for a more sensual feeling.

The Turned Kiss

If you want to tease your lover and make them feel gentleness and tenderness go for this type of kiss. This type of kiss is also perfect when you want to start foreplay with your partner. Also when you're making love slowly in a face-to-face standing or sitting position.

To perform this type of kiss, one of you, preferable the man turns up the face of his love by holding the chin and head. In that position, he then goes in slowly as your lips touch hers.

The Straight Kiss

When you kiss your love with your heads, you wouldn't be able to have so much of the tongue penetration. This kiss isn't to express an intense passion but a gentle way of showing affection and expression of desire. This type of kiss is recommended for new lovers.

To perform this type of kiss, let your lover sits on your laps and uses your hand to caress, fondle, her body, especially her back while kissing. Then as you go for the kiss, let your heads be angled only slightly, that it would seem almost straight. Then let your lips come in direct contact with each other and enjoy yourself.

Pressed Kiss

This type of kiss is more of an erotic prelude to kissing. It's sensual as you'd feel the contact of your lovers lips. There are two ways you can have this kiss with your lover.

The first method is when you are kissing your lover, and you press your lover's lower lips with force. This kiss expresses the degrees of passion you feel for your lover at that moment. And if you do it right, it can prelude to even more foreplay and clothes go off, and you know the rest.

For the second method, you use your lips to touch your loves lower lips first, then you go for a greatly pressed kiss. This other type of kiss is even more emotional than the first one, so you can choose any one of the two types of pressed kisses to show how much passion is in your heart.

Kissing the Upper Lips

This kissing from the teaching in Kama Sutra, Vatsyayana talks about a woman returning a man's kiss, making it clear that a woman can also initiate the kiss. This can also apply to other forms of lovemaking. So, women shouldn't feel afraid to make the first move.

To perform this kiss, as you kiss your lover's upper lips, she returns the kiss by kissing his lower lip. You can increase the sensuality of the kiss by kissing your partner's upper and lower lips in turn. And like most kisses, you and your lover can have it sitting, standing or lying down.

The Clasping Kiss

This type of kiss is the one where either the woman or man takes both the lips of the other between her or his lips. However, for the woman, you can only enjoy taking this kiss when your lover doesn't have a mustache. That way, you don't have to get all those hair in your mouth.

When you are enjoying this type of kiss with your lover and your lover uses his/her tongue to touch the tongue, teeth, or palate of your lover, it's called the fighting of the tongue. Generally, in clasping kiss, scrupulous oral hygiene is important.

A Young Girl's Kiss

The young girl's kiss is a type of kiss the Kama text recommend for lovers who are about to have sex for the first time. There are different types of young girl's kiss, and it's recommended that the kiss is done moderately and not to be continued for a long time.

The nominal kiss: to have this kiss like a girl, use your mouth to touch your love's own. But don't do the touching yourself, approach your lover closely, and he would do the touching himself.

The throbbing kiss: to have this kiss as a girl set your bashfulness aside touches the lips of her lover that is pressed into her mouth and with an object moves her lower lips but not the upper one.

The touching kiss: to have this kiss as the girl kiss your lover by using your tongue to touch his lips. As you close your eyes, place your hands on your lover's hands and enjoy the kiss.

Other ways to use kissing

Apart from the above-mentioned types of kissing, there are other ways you and your lover can engage in kissing. These different forms of kissing can be used for different purposes. Here are some examples of the different ways to use kissing.

Kissing that kindles love

Just like the name suggests, this kissing a woman can use to arouse her partner. She can use it to wake her partner up when she is feeling amorous. When she kisses him, she should look at his face while he sleeps. And she should kiss him passionately, softly and with desire. This type of kissing shows her intention and desires to her lover.

Kissing that awakens

In this type of kissing, lovers can quickly use it to rekindle the love they have for each other. A man can use this kissing on his lover. When a man comes home late in the night, for example, and he finds his lover asleep, he can then go to her and place a kiss on her. This kiss shows her his intention, and occasionally, the woman could even pretend to be asleep to wait for her lover to come home and kiss her this way.

Kissing that turns away

Now when your lover seems to be carried away, or his mind seems to be somewhere else, as a woman, you can use a kiss to turn his mind away. Perhaps you both just had a quarrel, or maybe he is attending a business or looking at something else, a kiss is perfect to bring his mind back to you.

Kissing the body

The lips and breasts are very sensitive parts of the body, and when touched with the mouth can bring lots of pleasure. In general. The closer you kiss your lover to the genitals, the more irresistible and intense the pleasure would be. The body should be kissed by both loves at the same time for more pleasure, especially around the foot to the head. The intensity at which you kiss the body should vary in terms of intense, moderate, pressed, or soft.

Breast kissing: when you want to kiss your lover's breast, be sure to apply it lightly to the fullness of the breast, as you gently suck and rub the nipples. You should pay special attention to the nipples because for many women; the nipple is a very powerful arousing point.

Kissing and licking: as lovers, you both should participate in kissing and licking. You should also pay special attention to areas like the inside thigh, the back of the knees, nipples, and breast. The greater you have self-control in delaying penetration, the richer the rewards when it finally occurs. You also combine the kissing and licking with a series of soft sensual strokes and kisses to enhance the effects of the kisses.

Biting

Loves can also engage in biting as a form of mouth play. Kama Sutra encourages it as it is an important part of the lover's repertoire. Biting can be done anywhere on the body and can range from playful nip to a more teasing than erotic, or it could be a sustained sucking that leaves a mark. Here are more details about biting you need to know as loves.

The biting of a boar

Lovers can use the biting of a boar when they want to leave a bite mark on their lover's shoulder. This bite is described as consisting of many board rows of marks near one another. It also usually have red intervals. You can make these markings on the shoulders as well as on the breasts which shows peculiar intense passion lovers have for themselves.

The broken cloud

This type of biting is described as consisting of unequal risings in a circle. This unequal circle is as a result of the space between the teeth. These type of biting is even best when you make a mark on the breast.

In addition to these two types of biting, there are eight other types of biting loves can engage in to show passion. These biting include the hidden bite, the swollen bite, and the point, the line of point, the coral and the jewel and the line of jewel.

Cunnilingus

Cunnilingus or oral sex where the virginal is being stimulated, and it is widely practiced in the modern world today. You should not run into trouble having this with your partner. Well, in some cases some partners feel somewhat irritated by the whole idea at first, but don't worry, you can talk them out of their irritation. And when you are able to talk them out of it, you can enjoy the sensation and special feeling of intimacy provided by oral sex.

Clitoral stimulation

Clitoral stimulation is a type of cunnilingus where the clitoris is gently stimulated with the lips or tongue. The clitoris is probably the most sensitive part of the woman's body, and as such, the clitoral stimulation would be exceedingly sensual. For this move, position yourself in a way that you can stroke your tongue over the shaft and head of her clitoris. If you like, your partner could be lying on her back, sitting or standing.

And if she's one of the many women that enjoy cunnilingus, she could experience a series or orgasm during the session. Stimulate the sides of the clitoris, run and you can go underneath too. Also, use your tongue to give feather-light strokes on the head of the clitoris and give it a flick underside of the shaft from the sides with the tip of your tongue.

Stimulating the perineum

To do this, let the woman open her legs widely, then you can get between them as you lick the perineum. The perineum is the area that lies between the vagina and the anus. This area is usually very rich in never endings and as such is very sensitive to touch. So use your tongue to touch, stroke and lick. When you stimulate the perineum properly, it can cause high arousal.

Fellatio

Unlike cunnilingus, that deals more of oral sex and mouth play on the virginal, fellatio is for male. It can be seen as mouth congress when the penis is stimulated until orgasm is experienced in most cases.

Licking the Penis

As a woman to start fellatio with your lover, start with licking his penis as though it were an ice cream cone. Then you can go ahead to hold the base of the penis with one hand and then use the blade of your tongue to lick the penis upward repeatedly. You can do this on one side and then on the other for maximum satisfaction.

Butterfly flick

The butterfly flick is another highly effective fellatio technique whereby you consistently flicker your tongue lightly on the ridge of the underside of your lover's penis. When you first start, you may need to hold the penis of your lover, but you would adapt to it in no time, and you would be able to perform it without having to use your hands. When you leave them as you caress and fondle the penis, pleases your lover even more.

Chapter 6: Kama Sutra Sex Positions Explained

I'm pretty sure this is the chapter you have long been waiting for, and as such I'd try my best to be as realistic with you as the positions can be. There are about a hundred sex positions explained in the Kama Sutra. But if I am to give you the full details of it, it would be somewhat too much for the budget of this book. However, who knows, I might write another book explaining only the sex position.

In that light, I would be explaining ten of the best sex position you and your partner can quickly try out to get the best sensual experience you've had in a while. So, without further ado, let's jump right into it.

1. The Pressing Position

The pressing position is one of the best and fulfilling positions you can try with your lover as it unfolds effortlessly from one embrace to a rhythm like lovemaking. This lovemaking is very sensual and can be used to connect with your partner deeply. And it is very easy to perform, and the best part is that both lovers would get to enjoy the lovemaking to the fullest.

To perform this lovemaking, lie your partner down on the bed after you must have had a series of foreplay. As she lies down on the bed, you can further go deeper with the foreplay by rubbing her breast, and nipples to arouse her further. Then you could go lower and play around her belly, and you approach her vagina. You could also place a kiss on her vagina, and a little clitoris stimulation would also help as you go into position for this lovemaking. Remember your lover is already lying flat on the bed back down.

Then spread both of her legs on either side of your waist and fix yourself in-between. Then move a bit forward and place your hands at her sides and lean softly on her. Then at this position, you can go for insertion. Upon entering her vagina, go easy, it would feel a bit tight at first, but after a couple of minutes, and with the right amount of vagina fluid from arousing her well, things should go a lot more smooth. The main should use his feet to apply pressure when making love in this position.

The woman could also grip her partner's thigh with her own and press it inwards to tighten her vagina to thrust his penis more thigh for more friction and pleasure which increases the sensation for both of you. Generally, this position is great because of the body contact around the limb, and belly region as well. Moreover, the more the partners roll around together as they press their limb together, the greater the sexual charge would be.

2. The Mare's Position

This is also another sex position from the Kama Sutra worth taking a look at as lovers. One of the advantages of this technique is that it can be done in various positions. And if the woman is those that contract during orgasm, then she could employ her vaginal muscles to squeeze her lover's penis as though she were milking the penis. This sex position is highly pleasurable, that is why I'm featuring it in this book.

To actually enjoy this position, as the man you can enjoy it in two positions – either lying back down. Or sitting with one hand on the bed for support. As usually, sex should always proceed after a series of foreplay. When emotions are high, and the two of you are really in the mood and want to dive into each other, then man should go to bed. As I said earlier, you can either take a seated position of back down position.

In that position, the woman crosses her legs over yours and faces the same direction you are facing. So, her back would be at your front. In that position, before you go for congress, you can further to do a little more foreplay, like kissing her back, playing with her hair, or squeezing the breast would not be a bad idea.

Then you can go for penetration as the man. On entering the vagina with your penis, it is best you take the lying down position at first as it helps reveals more of the penis for deeper penetration. As you penetrate, you can then sit up for more joyride. After some time enjoying this position with your partner, you feel very close to orgasm, you could take the sitting position as it helps to reduce the feeling of orgasm.

You could also help by stimulating her clitoris with your fingertips as you sit up. She could also do this herself, whichever you two lovebirds prefer would be just fine. One thing you both will enjoy again in this position is the skin contact because it is more like she is sitting on your lap. This sense alone can increase arousal to make the man have an orgasm in no time. Because you'd both feel the buttock bouncing on the laps making those clapping sounds turning both lovers on more. This position is enjoyable, and lovers should try it out.

3. The Turning Position

When couples are making love, alternating the position can help to make lovemaking more intense and sensual as well as increase closeness. The turning position is a perfect type of love, making that is perfect for this kind of feeling. To have the turning position lovemaking with your lover, have a couple of foreplay to make the woman end up with her back on the bed. Then as the man fix yourself in-between her legs and go for the insertion.

The lovemaking is more like the popular missionary lovemaking, but it comes with a twist. During lovemaking, the man can change position by lifting one of his legs and turn around without withdrawing from her. There are different ways the man can turn around in this position. There are about four different stages in this turning position.

The first stage is just like what I just explained above, the regular missionary position. The woman can caress and stroke the chest of her lover to give him more arousal, which can be a tricky maneuver. For the second stage, the man would lift his left leg and then his right leg to his lover's right leg and should not withdraw his penis from her vaginal.

The third stage involves the man moving both of his legs around, and this time, he does it without withdrawing his penis. He should make sure his body is at the right angle with his lover. Her legs also should be slightly apart as it would make it easier for him to keep his penis inside her vagina. And for the woman, she should lie back and enjoy the unusual angle of penetration. And the last fourth position is when he makes a complete 180-degree rotation in the sense that his body is between her legs one leg on either side of her shoulders. Navigating through these four stages of sex position is a bit difficult. But with practice, you would become a master in it in no time.

4. The Woman on Top Position

The woman on top is just like the turning position mentioned above, but this time around, the woman is on top of the man in this position. Again it comes in three different stages which the woman can use to vary the position while making love to make lovemaking more fun. To have this form of lovemaking with your partner, the man should lie back down.

The woman would then cross her legs one on either side of the man. As she sits on her lover, they should both lock their fingers together. Then as she balances herself on her partner's lap, the congress should happen. While making love in this position, then you both should switch positions. The first stage is when the woman is in the normal facing her lover while they make love.

The second stage is when she tilts both of her legs to her lovers left side or right side depending on whichever side she prefers. She could keep her legs together for more sensual feeling as her vaginal would be tight. Or she could spread her legs to make the vaginal a little bit more open. She can then steady herself by putting a hand on his knee and the other hand on his chest for support.

The third and last stage is when the woman makes a full complete rotation where she now backs the man. She can place her hand on her lover's leg as she rides him. She could make movements like she's tweaking on his penis to make the sex faster and more sensual.

5. The Yawning Position

The yawning position is somewhat popular, but not everyone gets it right. This lovemaking position starts with a man in a more-or-less kneeling position. However, his knees should be widely spread. Not too wide, though! It should just be the right width for the woman to fit. Then the woman lying with her back on the bed raises her thigh and parts them on either side of the man. Her legs might get tired with time, so she can press her legs against his side to make it easier to keep them up.

This position is pleasurable for both the man and the woman, but for the woman, it's all about getting the right thigh angle. Now, since the woman is lying down back on the bed, and the man on top (kneeling), pressing her thighs together, his side is an easy way to vary her thigh angle. Adjusting her thigh angle is also a way of varying the depth of penetration. Also, the barrier of the woman's thigh doesn't allow very deep penetration, but her clitoris gets much stimulation.

The man, on the other hand, should thrust himself forward gently against the woman's lower thigh for the penetration. He should also interlace his hands with the woman's hand to keep him up while penetrating. In general, this position is really erotic. Not to mention, her genitals are exposed, which turns the man on more. The helplessness she feels being on the bed in that locked position can also be a powerful turn on for both of them.

What you should note about this position is that her leg would feel a bit heavy with time since blood wouldn't flow much to her legs. So, don't use this position for a prolonged period. Also, since the man is somewhat resting on her hands, her hand would also feel tired at some point. Plus if you're a fan of fast sex, this position wouldn't really work for you. This position is for people who prefer a more gentle to a moderate speed of sex.

6. The Elephant Posture

This sex position is highly recommended as it is very sensual and comes with a lot of joy attached. This position is so powerful because there are lots of body contact involved in the position. Lovers who want to connect with each other deeply can have a fun time enjoying this position. To perform this position, very little is needed to know about from the right foreplay that would lead to this position.

To begin lovemaking in this position, start with the right foreplay that would make you get to your lovers back. Kissing her whole body round could be a great start. Or you can combine kissing her body with a little hair play and then find your way to her back. Kiss her shoulder and bend her over until she's lying down with her stomach, thigh, breast, and feet all touching the bed. In this position, you could go for a little massaging to stimulate her even more.

Massage her back, and go down a little to massage her buttocks. Massage her around her vagina and stimulate her clitoris until she fills wet on her vagina. Then you can go for the penetration, for the penetration, place your hands and either side of your lover and lean on her buttock a bit. Then like you, as you go for the penetration, pass your penis between her slightly parted legs and get into her vagina.

This sex position is very sensual as you would enjoy the feeling of her buttock around the penis, which is very pleasurable. The woman can intensify the sensation for both of you by pressing her thigh closely once the man is insider her to increase the feeling.

7. Level Feet Posture

This position is a type of Ananga Ranga way of lovemaking. This position can be a bit difficult to do and is not a position that can be enjoyed for a prolonged period of time. To perform this lovemaking, you need to find a way to end the foreplay with the woman back on the bed. But if you are a couple who love to have deep penetration, sex would definitely enjoy this type of lovemaking as the position reveals the vagina in a way that penetration can go deep.

To perform this lovemaking, with the woman is lying down, raise her legs up and place them on your shoulder. One leg on either side of her partner as she pushes herself closer towards his penis. Then the man supports her by holding her sides around her rib and then goes for the penetration. As he goes for the penetration, she could increase the pressure by closing her thing, which would make the penetration more pleasurable on his deep-plunging penis.

8. The Crab Embrace Position

As lovers, if you want a sex position that you can do for a very prolonged period, then this is perfect for you. The crab and embrace position is more of a side-by-side position in the sense that you and your partner are both lying down side by side facing each other. The penetration in this position would be deep. However, the man's movement would be restricted in a way. This sex position is very sensual as you can look deep into your lover's eyes as you make love and use your hands to caress each other. You both could even have a deep sensual kiss in-between the sex.

To perform this inviting and warm sex position, the man would lie right next to the woman and places one of his legs in-between her legs. In this lying position, he then goes for the penetration. And like I said earlier, the penetration movement wouldn't be much, so done expect too much movement. This position is also great, especially when you and your lover have been having sex for a prolonged time, and you are both tired but still passionate to have sex.

When the sex is going on in this position, you can add loving caresses to the mix. Use your free hand to caress each other's face, torso, arms, thighs, and buttocks. Again, the leg position is also important in this sex position, so make sure you put your uppermost leg over his body and rest your knee back to his hip.

9. The Rainbow Arch Position

It is never a bad idea to try something new, and this sex position is definitely going to be something new in your archive. This sex position is somewhat difficult, but when you get a hold of the idea of the position, it will come in a lot easier. This sex position is a side by side sec position, and the posture has an unusual angle for penetration, which has a very sensational feeling attached.

To perform this sex position with your lover, you and your lover are to both lies down flat on the bed. As the woman lies down, she is to raise one of her legs up sure that the man can fix himself in-between her opened legs. The man should fix himself, in-between her legs in such a way that his face goes to the back of the woman while his legs come to her front. Then as he goes for the penetration, he holds her shoulder to make the movement easier. She can hold his leg for support, so she doesn't move too much while the man applies more pressure for the lovemaking.

10. Driving the Peg Home

This is a standing posture sex position. It might involve some strength from the man's side, but it is definitely worth the strength. Strength is needed in the sense that the man would need to lift the woman up for the penetration. So, for lovers to enjoy this sex position, the man needs to be strong so that he can thrust his penis satisfactorily while bearing the weight of his partner. However, great care is needed because his member is very vulnerable to damage in this position so he should take great care when making love with this position.

To perform this position. The man should lift the woman and support her up by holding her buttocks. Then she is to thrust her legs at either side of her lover but to hold on to her lover's waist tightly while she holds his shoulder. She is also to keep her back straight as she leans against the wall.

Chapter 7: Before and After Sex

Now that you have all you need to know about the Kama Sutra, it is now that time where we are to talk about what is to be done before and after sex. Well, in summary, you should do those things that increase your passion before sex and those things that keep the amusement after sex. If you are having sex with your partner, there should be something that should be done before and after depending on your relationship with your lover.

The things you are to do varies, for example, if you don't want to risk having a baby after the sex, or you're scared of sexually transmitted diseases, which is very common in this modern world. So, in order to avoid stories that touch, it is in everyone's interest that lovers take the necessary precautions.

What to do before sex by having a safer sex

When having sex, it is very important that you bring the risk involved to the minimum. If you completely trust your partner, then there is no need for this safer sex. But if on the other hand, you just got a new partner and you're considering having sex, it is the only saver to protect yourself. Or at least it is important you have protected sex unite you are sure your lover is clear. Probably when you both have gone for a checkup, or a test, only then can you fully relax your mind of the safety of your partner.

There are two ways I am going to be talking about in which players can indulge in for safer sex. These two safer sex methods include non-penetrative sex and the use of condoms. Let us look into these two a bit to see what we can learn from them regarding safety before sex.

Non-Penetrative Sex

This is a type or method of having sex which is very sensitive to the lovers, but there is no penetration involved. Non-penetrative sex could include applying dry kissing, stroking, massage and embracing or a combination of any one of them. When you do not want to lose the closeness you have with your partner yet you do not want to risk any sexually transmitted infection, then you can both indulge in non-penetrative sex.

Mutual masturbation can also be a great way of having non-penetrative sex. But to be extra safe, make sure no vaginal fluid or semen comes in contact with your hands in case of any cuts, open sores, or abrasion on your hand.

Using Condoms

Using a condom is one of the safest ways to have sex without having to go through all the trouble of worrying too much. The major objective of using a condom is to interrupt your body and your lover's body fluid like semen or vaginal fluid from coming in contact during sex. Again condoms could also reduce the sensation a man feels his penis during lovemaking.

To use a condom, carefully remove it from the packet and squeeze out the air in the condom. Then hold the tip of the forefinger and thumb and with slow sensuous movement slide the condom down your partner's penis. And if your partner is not circumcised, gently push the foreskin back before unrolling the condom on his penis.

What to do after sex by prolonging the mood

After lovemaking, you and your partner could still keep the vibes going by engaging yourself to one or more activities that would keep the mood up. A lot of couples have confirmed that after having sex, they find it easier to communicate with each other. Some couples find it easier to talk about things while having sex, and others prefer having a conversation after having sex. In a case where you don't intend to continue having sex, but the man had, and orgasm but the woman didn't get the opportunity to reach climax, the ideal thing for the man to do is to masturbate her until she reaches orgasm.

Rekindle the excitement

Rekindling the excitement is a way lovers could spark up the mood to continue having sex. For example, a woman can renew the erection of her lover by gently fondling his testicles. She could use one hand to slide the other up and down his penis. Another scenario is enhancing the arousal of the man's penis. To further enhance the arousal, she could brush the head of his penis by making featherlight circular strokes with her hand.

As a man, you can rekindle the excitement by helping your lover get to orgasm. This is exceedingly important in a case where your partner was not able to reach a climax during lovemaking. Or a man could do this for his lover if she wants more orgasm, but you are not ready for more love again. You can help her by using your fingers to stimulate the clitoris. Gently run the tip of your finger along the underside and each side and on top of her vagina as you stimulate.

Sustaining the harmony

A lot of lovers don't want to give up the warm glow they get from making love by going to sleep of turning over, or by doing anything that is intellectually, or physically demanding. Some loves love to follow lovemaking with a gentle sensual massage, while others prefer to lie down quietly in each other's arms. In all, there can sustain harmony by engaging in other things. Things like eating together or any other undemanding activity would work just fine.

Chapter 8: The Benefits of Kama Sutra

Kama Sutra is a very wonderful text that teaches us a lot about sex. As lovers, it is important that you take the teachings of Kama Sutra seriously so that you would be able to create a more stable relationship. As you already know, the Kama Sutra goes far deeper than talking about sex. Although the book talks about sex positions, the book also makes emphasis on ways of having a satisfying sex life. Following the Kama Sutra teachings, you stand a chance to become more educated about male and female. Here is some truth about the Kama Sutra you probably didn't know.

1. Kama Sutra values empowering women

Despite all what our modern-day society keeps preaching about women and sexuality, Kama Sutra has a different view on this subject matter. Kama Sutra suggests that a woman needs to study the different forms of sex before she gets married. When a woman understands the different forms of sex, she would be a better mate and would be more desirable by her man. So, the Kama Sutra encouraging women and empowering them is one of the biggest benefits you stand to gain from the book.

2. Kama Sutra makes a clear classification of a man's penis

Also, the Kama Sutra made mention of the size of a man's penis and that it matters when choosing a mate. There are three types of man penis by Kama Sutra – the bull, horse, and hare. Kama Sutra also made mention of different sizes of woman's vagina, and that a perfect match of the vagina size and penis sizes would result in a good sexual experience. In a case where you are married to a woman where the man's penis size and the woman's vaginal size is not a perfect match, then such couple would experience a little setback in the different sexual positions they can try out. So, thanks to Kama Sutra, we can make the right choice regarding the penis and vaginal sizes to enjoy a full sensual experience.

3. Kama Sutra also emphasizes on living a healthy life and well-balanced one

Kama Sutra is also a book that talks about tips on how to live a healthy life. The Kama Sutra encourages that a man and a woman should embrace cleanliness which would, in turn, boost their health. A man, for instance, should shave his beard on a regular basis, and take his bath and eat healthily, and the same applies to a woman too. She should bread her hair and shave as well. Couples could also try mutual grooming.

4. Kama Sutra talks about enticing and approaching women

The Kama Sutra also talks about interesting tips a man can use to entice and approaching a woman. This tip helps men to know how to touch and caress a woman in other to express their desire when they want to have sex. When a man knows these various tips and how to use them, he will find it easier to get his message over to the woman. The tips of how to entice and approach a woman further move on to touching and embracing.

5. Kama Sutra talks about eight different types of embrace

There are different types of embrace from the Kama Sutra. It further tells us that there are up to eight different types of embrace which can be used for different purposes. Because of Kama Sutra teaching, we now know how to apply the various types of embrace. And on applying the right type of embrace at the right moment would set the right mood in motion. So, rather than keeping all your emotions inside, you can now use the various teaching from Kama Sutra about embrace to seduce and lure your lover into that perfect love zone.

6. Kama Sutra teaches about kissing

There are different forms of kissing too. Kama Sutra also teaches that a woman should feel too shy about a kiss. We all know that a man in most cases is the ones that initiate the kiss, but a woman should not feel shy to be the one to start the kiss first. There are also different types of kiss that partner can use to deeply connect with each other at particular points in your relationship. Like a type of kissing couples can engage in when walking on a lonely street. There are also different types of kiss that lovers can engage in when they want to make love.

7. Kama Sutra is divided into a set of 64 acts

Contrary to the belief that the Kama Sutra doesn't have a list of sex position howbeit lovemaking that includes penetration is divided into 64 acts. This acts explains the different ways couples can have sex to enjoy the maximum pleasure from sex. To have the best sex, you have to combine it with stimulating desire, and engaging in an embrace, caressing, kissing, biting, slapping, moans, oral sex, and everything in-between.

8. Kama Sutra recommends that your scratch your partner

There are different types of scratch you can have with your partner. With this knowledge Kama Sutra provide us, we can add a twist to lovemaking without loved ones. Moreover, leaving scratch marks on your lover's body can help keep the fire burning for each other even when your lover is not close to you.

9. Kama Sutra recommends that your woman lover should reach orgasm first

When making love with our loved once, Kama Sutra suggests that the woman should be the first to have an orgasm. This point is valid because of the extreme exhaustion a man feels after having an orgasm, whereby he wouldn't be able to proceed with sex at least not immediately. So, in other to have great sex, the woman should be the first to have an orgasm before the man allows himself to have an orgasm.

10. Kama Sutra also talks about a woman's sex as being more than just sex penetrations

In Kama Sutra, there is more to sex than penetration for a woman. To a woman, the whole act is sensual, but to a man reaches orgasm at the end of the intercourse. Most men think that making a woman have an orgasm is their ultimate act, but a woman needs both sexual and physiological pleasure to be able to satisfy her urge. Thanks to Kama Sutra, many men who were getting this concept wrong have been able to make adjustments.

Chapter 9: How to Apply Everything you've Learnt about Kama Sutra

Now that you have completed reading this book, you may wonder what is next? Well, what happens next is to apply all you've learned from the Kama Sutra. There is no point in learning something like the Kama Sutra without applying it. What was given in this book are all practicable most of which are information gotten from friends and families, personal experience, and from various researches? So, feel completely free to try out any sex position that caught your attention.

When you can successfully apply everything you have learned about Kama Sutra from this book, you would experience a bit change in your sexual life. Now, if you are feeling a bit confused on how to apply Kama Sutra, don't worry I've got you covered. I've put together five easy to learn a step-by-step process you can follow to apply Kama Sutra to your love life successfully.

1. Approach your lover

The first and most important thing you need to do is first to make an approach. If you do not make a harmless approach, you would never know what your partner loves, and what they don't. There are different ways you can approach your lover about the whole idea of the Kama Sutra. Many people often prefer to just come out clean with the whole idea of the Kama Sutra, which normally works for them. They often come back with a smile on their face that by simply talking with their partner was all they needed.

However, it isn't everyone that is endowed with this gift. So, if you know deep down your lover would have second thoughts about the Kama Sutra, don't bother approaching her with a conversation of the Kama Sutra, rather show it to her. Make her feel a difference in you, more like a new you.

2. Make an Attempt

Next step you are to take after deciding what approach you want to use to lure your partner into Kama Sutra, is to make an attempt. Now, this step is very crucial as you wouldn't want to rush things a little too much. So, start with the basics. Don't attempt with her with difficult sex positions; in fact, try to avoid the sex positions when you start. Keep your attempts to foreplay and kissing.

You don't want to speak your lover or make them feel disgusted by the Kama Sutra because they are not used to it. And you know what they say about the first impression, it last longer. So, make sure you give your lover a really memorable first impression. Make her feel those sensations, touch her at those sensitive points we talked about the erogenous zones. Play around with her, make her laugh, make her feel something so sensual that she'd have to close her eyes and open her mouth because she can't hold it in altogether.

3. Seduce

When you're making the right attempt, and it seems to be working, that is just perfect because what you're going to do next is to go for the seduction part. This could be the part where you add a little massage to the mix. Try massaging her with oil, or better still dry but make it a full naked both massage. Then as you massage her, occasionally go towards her buttocks, go towards her vaginal area, and stimulate the clitoris from time to time. And don't forget also to rub and massage the breast as well.

For the man, be sure to massage his penis and around his balls, a blow job too would go a long way in causing arousal. Seduction should be very sensual and filled with so much emotion. If you want to do it right, make sure the environment is conducive. We've spoken about making the environment perfect, so be sure to employ it the right way. Make the room warm when it is cold outside, or cold wand well aerated when it is warm outside.

4. Go for any of the sex positions you've learned

When you have finally groomed your lover to the extent that all they can think about is sex with you, then you're halfway there. At this point, this is when you are going to apply the best sex position you've learned. Also, don't start with something too difficult. Go for something very simple, something very pleasurable, and something that is more of pleasure than of a sex position itself.

As soon as you go for in penetration, be sure to take things slowly at first. Don't also forget to stimulate other parts of her body as you continue to make love to her. Then feel free to change sex position from time to time as you progress in love.

5. Try an after sex fun

Last but not least, after sex, you can engage in a conversation with your lover. Ask him or her what they like about sex, so you can know where to shift and make an adjustment. With time, you'd only get better and making romantic hot crazy sex with your lover.

Conclusion

The world waits for no man. When you have a plan for your life, especially a life-changing program, do not procrastinate. There are more things you stand a chance to win. So, no matter the challenge you face on the road, always keep pushing forward. You might try to attempt Kama Sutra, but your lover keeps turning the idea down over and over. In such a case, don't give up, things can get very challenging, but with perseverance, you will achieve great things.

"Go for it now. The future is promised to no one" –
Wayne Dyer

www.ingramcontent.com/pod-product-compliance
Lightning Source LLC
Chambersburg PA
CBHW030916080526
44589CB00010B/331